ROCKET

FUEL

*The High Octane in Your DNA
That Can Propel You to Greatness*

PHILLIP TOMLINSON, M.S.

I didn't have to think very hard about this.

You see, when my mother gently and lovingly tugged at my heartstrings and said, among other things, "You should write a book!" she earned this mention.

But she also had you in mind, because she believed there's someone to whom this could make a real difference.

If I absolutely believed there was no one who would open this book, there'd be no point to the chapters that follow.

YOU are, therefore, part of my inspiration. If I can make even a small difference to just you, it would be worth it.

So, yes, while I dedicate this to my mother, Icodel Tomlinson, who remains a big part of my inspiration, THIS ONE IS ALSO FOR YOU!

Thank you for turning the page.

CONTENTS

FOREWORD

ROCKET FUEL IS AN honest, back-to-basics blueprint. Phil's inspiring narrative is, in many ways, our story.

The way he weaves his personal journey into a world of innocence we all once inhabited is special. I hope you recognize the genius here.

His easy-to-read account is sure to get you thinking. I couldn't help but do just that. His football references in particular had me thinking back to my gridiron days.

One reference, for example, "inches make champions," couldn't be a more basic truth.

I can definitely relate. This is a concept that defines not just any good football team but the road to success in general.

Fighting for inches is where it begins, because if we can do that, we'll be prepared to fight for more. It's how we snatch victory from the jaws of defeat.

I know because this is the mindset that has always fired me up. It had me turning inches into more, and it paid off big—from back when, as a skinny seventeen-year-old kid, I was sought after by college football giants like Notre Dame, USC, Yale, Penn State, and Ohio State.

It's the mindset that led to big getting bigger when, as an academic all-American tight end, I drafted into the NFL, played alongside some of the greatest athletes on the planet, and, ultimately, became a double Super Bowl winner, catching two key passes during the winning touchdown drive in Super Bowl XXIII.

This may not define greatness, because greatness can be defined in many ways. So, this book nudges you into taking a look at yourself, while reuniting you with a blueprint that can usher you through the doorway to realizing your true potential.

Phil does this with a truly human touch because, as he tells his own story, he revisits the ups and downs of parenthood and takes you through the rich narratives of the streets of New York. Insightfully, he leads you down a path that shows how vulnerability can be a path to winning.

I've admired Phil's easy-going yet take-no-prisoners winning attitude ever since meeting him some sixteen years ago. I've benefited from his expertise and, similarly, I'm sure, as you read *Rocket Fuel*, you'll encounter a process that enriches you as well.

John E. Frank, MD/Plastic Surgeon

Winner, Super Bowl XIX and Super Bowl XXIII

INTRODUCTION

HE WAS HARD TO miss, being so tall and rangy. I placed him perhaps in his sixties. And as he climbed aboard the New York City Transit bus I was riding, I noticed he had a significant limp.

"Going to school?" he said in his pleasant Southern drawl, engaging my three-year-old twins. Then, pulling up one leg of his pants, he exposed the reason for his limp: a metal prosthesis. "Don't be out in the street doing what you shouldn't be doing," he cautioned, directing his soft gaze at my wide-eyed kids. "I was hit by a car doing something I shouldn't be doing, and, see? You'll pay for it for the rest of your life." His explanation had no bitterness.

This was a *magic moment*, inspired by adversity.

He had the perfect motivation, and I couldn't help but think he'd supplied this caution from the heart many times before.

This incident reminded me of my own motivation for writing this book, which also sprang from adversity that initiated a teaching moment for me.

You see, while I lay in a hospital bed without the use of my legs, I began to see things in a way I never had before. My disability inspired me to pass on some valuable lessons, as I picked myself up—going from being unable to walk up even one rung of stairs to bounding up eighteen flights at a full sprint.

The lessons I'm talking about would be helpful in any endeavor in which you would like to find success. But, as a fitness coach, I've seen how a lack of motivation, for whatever reason, can keep so many of us sitting on the fence as our health disappears further and further into the distance.

So, yes, in alluding to my own experience, I am talking about *reclaiming health*. You see, in doing what we can to find our best health, we will also find our best life.

But this book is not about me, because, in the next chapters, you will come to recognize an intimate part of yourself that, like most of us, you have quite likely taken for granted: that *high-octane rocket fuel* that has worked like magic for you from the very beginning.

It's that magical part of you that, unfortunately for so many, has taken its leave.

In reintroducing you to that magic, this book will chart the way to a forgotten blueprint that can power you to greatness.

CHAPTER 1

A Win from Taking a Walk to Nowhere

I REMEMBER IT as if it were yesterday. I was in a hospital bed on the morning after, only a few hours removed from surgery. I lay on my back with ice packs beside me.

That morning, the physical therapy team stopped by to tell me I'd be taking a walk, with a little help—with the aid of a walker.

As they helped me out of bed onto the walker, it suddenly hit me. *That* was what caused the sinking feeling in my gut, the flushness in my face, and those sweaty palms.

Fright!

That's what it was.

I'd be going nowhere that day, not with my legs dragging, lifeless, behind me.

And, for a moment, I thought, "This is it. I'll never walk again!"

Then, unexpectedly, my brain made a connection. Because, you see, our lives are made up of stories that interconnect. We may not immediately see how those stories interconnect, but they do in some way. And sometimes, maybe even years later, we're amazed at how they do, especially when events lead down the least-expected path.

I have now written this book precisely because of one of those stories and its interconnections.

Research has it that eighty-one percent of Americans would like to write a book, but only three percent ever do.

I, too, have always wanted to write a book. I remained mired among the eighty-one percent for long stretches of time, however, because I had lost the kid in me. I would get cold feet, be less than courageous, and, frankly, oftentimes throwing in the towel.

It's been said that lost time can never be regained. Right alongside that maxim are lost opportunities—gone up in smoke, never to return.

While my prolonged procrastination may have amounted to throwing in the towel, however, my mind never really let go:

> There was a book in me somewhere.

When it came about the way it did, I thought of another age-old adage: Be careful what you ask for!

If you had told me I would have to lie in a hospital bed without the use of my legs in order to be able to write a book, I would surely have said, "No, thank you!" Especially since, as a martial artist, moving my body in powerful and unusual ways was as effortless as breathing.

Going from this ease to requiring a walker was not ever my idea of progress. But, in a curious way, this was winning—just not in the way I imagined winning to be.

And, as you might expect, I never recognized it for what it was until the idea for this book came about, because I could not have written this particular book without having gone through the hardship I described.

I had to pay a price to win.

Adversity can be that fuel that drives you to find answers—to see things in ways you never would have, otherwise.

That is what happened on the day I discovered I no longer had legs under me.

I took a walk to nowhere and came up with a win somewhere, when stories interconnected and the journey toward writing this book began.

CHAPTER 2

Envisioning My Stairway to Heaven

"NOT TODAY," said the therapist. "We just wanted to see what you could do."

What could I do at that point? Nothing, it turned out. And a walker wasn't going to be even a little help.

I needed a lot more than a little help, which sent my head into a tailspin. But while the feeling of helplessness can reduce you to spaghetti, it can also trigger resolve.

Not long after I had that sinking feeling that I'd never be able to walk again, something popped into my mind. I did a sudden 180. Just like that!

"Hell, yeah!" I thought.

Of the 2,500 to 3,300 thoughts that pass through our minds each hour in rapid succession, on this day desperation was the reason why one in particular hovered like a bright light in front of me.

I suddenly recalled a feel-good story that demonstrated, in an instant, no mountain is too high, especially when it comes to kids. And once they've decided to make the trek, it's a done deal.

Innate curiosity can make things interesting and, well, sometimes a little nervy. Even more so when that mountain is a steep staircase and the kid attempting to climb it hasn't yet fully learned to walk.

But one parent's worry may turn out to be a kid's stairway to heaven, which is exactly the way it turned out on the day I watched little Lindsay Guerrero, just over one year old, attempt to climb the stairway of a random Brooklyn brownstone.

Of course, she tried it the conventional way—by simply walking up. There was just one problem: Her legs were barely long enough or strong enough to handle each step without mishap.

So, I anxiously took her hand. But, as I would soon discover, she had a different approach in mind, one that didn't include me.

She let out a shriek and quickly yanked her hand away. Then she did what any kid does in that sort of a pinch: she resorted to the next best thing—all fours.

It worked like a charm. Slowly but surely, she motored all the way to the top until she stood, triumphant, on her own Iwo Jima. Then, waving her arms, she again shrieked for my help to take her back to the foot of the stairs.

And because kids will be kids, she did this several times over, climbing her way, having fun, and ensuring a little bodily development at the same time.

It was with this memory that my own recovery began. The moment also placed me on a path to discovery. Recalling that story while in my hospital bed helped me envision my own stairway to heaven.

CHAPTER 3

Turning a Loss into a Win

HAVE YOU EVER BEEN so shocked by something that you became week-kneed, like the life was about to drain out of you?

That's how I felt after the MRI that confirmed my legs could no longer carry me, let alone support me, to perform with the speed, efficiency, and skill I had, after my thirty-plus years of martial arts training had transformed my body into a highly tuned machine.

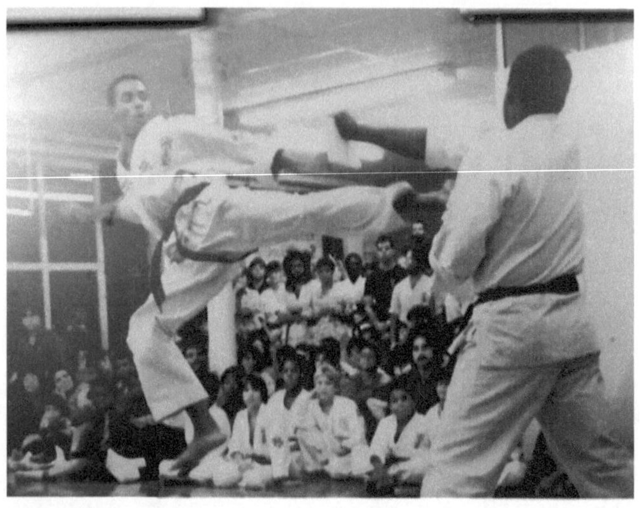

Years of martial arts training had transformed my body into a high-level machine

What really sickened me, however, was when the doctor said, "I'm seeing from the x-rays that you have cysts on the top of your femur. It's bone against bone."

I needed no clarification. I knew enough to understand he meant the cartilage—the shock absorbers—in my hips were gone. This news was a kick in the gut.

Although things in my legs had been souring for some time before the doctor made his diagnosis, I never expected this. And with my years of martial arts training structured around building a fighting spirit, this was a particularly hard truth to learn.

For a while, my spirit was crushed. This was an opponent like no other.

To the uninformed, a well-trained martial artist may be seen simply through the lens of fighting. In reality, however, the larger fight is with one's self, in terms of upholding the true spirit of training.

It is that spirit that will, oftentimes, guide the practitioner to walk away from a physical fight. But not this time.

It may not have been a fight with kicks and punches, but it was, for me, still a physical fight. And there was no walking away from this one!

In fact, it wouldn't be long before I would not be able to walk without simply ambling or using a cane. It was that bad. Then, bad decided to go postal one evening, as I exited an apartment building.

My hips and legs became so paralyzed with pain, I momentarily froze. I tried desperately to hold on to my pride by pretending to forget something. I hesitated and pretended to ponder, so as not to alert the doorman that I was in trouble.

But I was gripped with fear by what was happening to my body. It took all the willpower I could muster to fight through intense pain and nonchalantly walk out the door. Then, I turned the corner and, once out of sight, grabbed onto a nearby fence for support before bursting into tears, though less from pain and more from having lost the wind in my sails.

"Jesus!" I said in disbelief. "I can't walk!"

Yes, my own mind, which generated that desperation, is the same one that flies through those thousands of thoughts per hour. The amazing thing is this powerful agency can work in ways that are simply incredible, when adversity pushes us to the brink.

That baby climbing the stairs of a brownstone is a vivid reminder of that. She may not have been able to climb the stairs while standing up, but she would not be deterred. She turned a walk to nowhere into a win.

For the most part, we think we should avoid adversity at all cost. But the truth is, we cannot.

However, if we call it "friend" and embrace it wholeheartedly, we'll find it is that fuel that will light our path to the stairway to heaven.

CHAPTER 4

Stairway to Heaven

HAVE YOU EVER SEEN an opportunity that spells pure delight and inspires the kind of excitement that awakens a kaleidoscope of butterflies within?

I have. And I can tell you firsthand this was one of those life-changing opportunities.

I was one guy among dozens of morning commuters who regularly exited the train at New York City's East 64th Street Lexington Avenue subway line.

When you get off at this stop, if you so desire, you could be on your way to heaven... Well, heaven on earth. But first, every traveler faces one very steep escalator and then another, each seemingly on its way to the skies instead of merely to street level.

On either side of those two escalators are two sets of stairs that, needless to say, when it comes to going up, are rarely traveled. Actually, they are so steep that just gazing up those stairs is enough to make you nauseous.

So, they are hardly ever navigated, except when it came to this one guy among the dozens of other commuters, because—that's right! You guessed it! He never took the escalators. Yes, I never took the escalators.

Instead, I staked my claim to those pieces of real estate no one else cared for. That was how those two stairways became mine, at least for the time it would take me to sprint up one and then the other without skipping a beat. By the time I reached street level, my heart was seemingly about to beat out my chest, and I had been firing on all cylinders up the stairway to heaven.

I embraced adversity as a friend, which not only rewarded me mightily but had me wanting a lot more. It wasn't long after that "more" had me awash in a kind of elation that left me momentarily emotional.

Suddenly, I was really walking on air.

That is the feeling I had one day as I looked up from the foot of the very impressive Kyoto Station "Daikaidan" Grand Stairway in Japan. My eyes were moist. In a painful way, I was left with this serious reminder: *Never take things for granted!*

Simply put, I felt lucky that day. I recalled how I had struggled to use that walker with my feet dragging behind me. But, as the Kyoto Station "Daikaidan" Grand Stairway beckoned, those butterflies in my stomach set off a thumping excitement, which fired me up enough to run up that stairway three times in rapid succession.

Yes, this was sweetness, indeed! Because, before I staked my claim to those Lexington Avenue staircases or shed a tear at the bottom of Kyoto Station "Daikaidan" Grand Stairway, I had been that baby again, learning to walk. And I couldn't even make it up two rungs of stairs.

I had to take true baby steps after I had major double-hip surgery to repair those arthritic hips. Yet, with exhilaration, I soon found how two rungs became a full flight of stairs. Eventually, I could take an incredible eighteen flights at a full sprint, and then, well, there I was, with pulse-pounding excitement, at the foot of the Grand Stairway, a spot where, since 1998, teams of runners dashed up its 171 steps, over seventy meters, in an annual spring event.

For me, climbing the Grand Stairway was a triumph of massive proportions. But my rehabilitation, in mind and body, was to continue, after I was blessed in spectacular fashion on one unforgettable, fateful day in October.

CHAPTER 5

Armed but Hardly Ready

"THIS IS IT," I thought, as I walked into an appliance store one October day. While I wasn't sure I'd end up making the best buy, I needed to come close, at least, in the short time I had.

The next day would be *big,* and I couldn't afford any screwups.

Simply put, there would be no do-overs. If I missed my chance the screw up would be monumental and emblazoned in my mind forever. In fact, the disappointment would carry well beyond just me, to include nearly all of my family members. Things had been a little hectic up until this point. I hadn't even made a little time to do some research before heading over to, hopefully, make my best buy.

As I stepped off the elevator on the basement level of the store, I looked around and thought, "Where the hell do I start?"

Frankly, I felt overwhelmed. Even more so when I saw all those camera displays, knowing I had a relatively short time to make a decision and be on my way.

I'll admit, for the enormity of the occasion, I really should have done this much, much earlier. My mind launched into a back-and-forth:

"I can't believe it! You did it again! What the hell is wrong with you?"

The "it" I was referring to was that I should have made this trip well in advance. But I do know about procrastination. For example, I risked not finishing graduate school by foolishly writing my master's thesis the night before it was due. All sixty-four pages!

Because, among other things, it leaves you no room for error, procrastination can be a real killer. Yes, you'll eventually crash and burn!

Anyway, as my internal back-and-forth trailed off, I began to focus on the task at hand, jolted by the realization I had only a few hours to familiarize myself with the camera of my choice.

It was D-Day, and I had better be ready to bring my best photography. At this point, I needed a good, user-friendly shooter.

It took me about a minute of browsing to make the decision I'd be better off placing my trust in the expertise of a salesperson to help me achieve this outcome. By the time I exited the store, I was armed but hardly ready. The truth is, for me, this was a first. And I had nothing to compare to the upcoming day.

CHAPTER 6

D-Day: That Day in October

THIS WAS REALLY what it means to have a front-row seat!

It was not at all like the day a friend gave me two of the choicest seats to a New York Knicks game, a few rows behind number-one Knicks fan, Spike Lee. As the Knicks made their entry to a base-thumping, ear-splitting musical backdrop, the excitement was palpable. Cameras started going off.

While that was quite a rush, inspired no less by the NBA's most valuable team, it paled in comparison to where I was now sitting.

To be sure, this was no game.

There was an audience of just one.

Me.

Some forty-five minutes before, I had been ushered inside. I awaited the grand entrance, camera in hand, and experienced a pulse-pounding anxiety as I watched all the preparation. Some experiences are forever etched into your memory and entire being. Even as I write this account, I can feel the same body-chilling tingle I did on that October day.

Then, suddenly, the *moment* arrived.

My heart raced as I readied my camera.

The stars were about to make their grand entry.

There would not be a phalanx of cameras going off, like on that day at the Knicks game. **Just my own. I had to capture perhaps the best, but definitely the most consequential shots I would ever take.**

Then it happened!

I can't tell you what I was thinking, because maybe I wasn't. But I do remember blurting out, "*Oh My God!*"

And from then on, my finger did the talking as I fired away.

This was welcomed stress. With adrenalin and cortisol at their peak, my stomach butterflies flew in perfect formation, hardwiring me for efficiency.

I saw her first. And what an entry it was!

She had her hands up, fists clenched in front of her face like a fighter, and her high-pitched voice erupted triumphantly. Then, about a minute later and no less dramatically, the tenor arrived, waving his legs around in a 180-degree split, as if conducting a chorus.

My giddy excitement kept me shooting, breathless.

But, as I welcomed my daughter, Aiko, and my son, Kiichi, on that momentous October day of their birth, I couldn't help but think something that has been said forever and ever and probably in as many languages as exist. And I'm willing to bet, no matter what language you speak, you, too, have heard it said: *Children are a blessing.*

Yes, and though I've heard it many times, this idea permeated my entire being on that day in October, through my own adversity. I had been granted a front-row seat to rediscovering a big truth that often eludes us somewhere along our journey of life.

This book is about rediscovering that truth, because, whether or not you're a parent, you, too, have had unique access from "the very beginning." This is truth that can truly inspire greatness.

CHAPTER 7

Opening the Door to Greatness

SOMETIMES, WE TAKE a lot for granted. We may never even give a thought to the many things that actually go right for us and move us through each day.

It has been said we should learn to appreciate what we *have* before time makes us appreciate what we *had*. Sometimes that requires a nudge or a push.

I had a painful experience some years back, after completing my master's program. (Yes! That same master's degree that nearly went up in smoke due to my procrastination!)

And with an attitude that translated into, "World, here I come," I started out being sure of this: I would take the job market by storm, especially since my master's degree was from one of world's most reputable universities.

So, almost immediately and with brash confidence, I began the task of sending out résumés. Then came the interviews. One after the other, they piled up.

Weeks turned into months, and months turned into more than a year. In fact, I hadn't taken the job market by storm, and the disappointment was crushing. I sank into the doldrums.

Then, that inner voice started to play tricks on me. It informed me at every turn that I was an empty shell, someone who just couldn't make the grade, so I couldn't be like all those other people.

This was when I really drank the Kool-Aid, because it was the specter of "those other people" that turned things deeply irrational. I felt like I was in an episode of *The Twilight Zone*.

Whenever I ventured outside, I just knew "those other people," with their attaché cases and smart business suits, were all looking at me. They, too, seemed to know I couldn't make the grade, and I had no patience for their perceived disdain. So, I stayed inside, to hide from the world.

Of course, that wasn't much help, because I couldn't hide from myself. To borrow a line from an episode of *The Twilight Zone*, "How do you escape when you have nowhere to go?"

Then I read something that showed me where to go. It urged me to really pay attention and keep a written record of all the positive things around me.

Yes, a drowning man grasps at straws. I ventured back outside, after having agreed to a two-month experiment.

Things were finally turned on their head after a small gesture of kindness.

As I rushed into the subway one afternoon, a train about to pull into the station. I reached for my MetroCard only to be frustrated: insufficient fare. I had that sinking feeling of going nowhere, which you likely recognize.

Then, out of nowhere, came a teen with his MetroCard in hand to usher me through the turnstile!

The more I kept an eye out for these positive moments, the more I encountered them. Yes, I began to see I actually had more than I thought, if I really took the time to appreciate life. I found that the universe does conspire to help us in a multitude of ways.

You see, it's not about whether we lose. It's about how we move to open the door to greatness by applying what we've learned. That is when, in a curious way, losing is winning.

Yes, a drowning man will do what it takes to stay afloat and preserve his sanity.

The determination it takes is noteworthy, but this mindset adjustment allows us to clear out all the cobwebs.

CHAPTER 8

Boom!

THEY WILL CATCH your attention and cause you to pause for a moment. Then your heart may beat a little faster, because something has touched a nerve.

They may cause you to cry, because you recognize a part of you—the part that needs a lift. That's when they make you think: think about where you are and force you to confront yourself. They inform you you've been throwing your hands up in the air and giving up.

Then, your emotions get the better of you. Your body begins to heat up, because a mindset adjustment is on its way. You swallow hard, because this is the beginning of a confrontation—a confrontation with yourself.

But facing and confronting our problems is not easy. So, we resist starting to do it.

Just for a moment, I'd like you to keep in mind the "they" I began talking about, and allow me, as a fitness coach, to use what's very familiar to me as an example of this resistance to starting to tackle a problem by confronting ourselves.

If you are overweight or out of shape, you may resist starting—resist doing anything about it, even though you know it threatens your health. Why? Because confronting yourself is not easy.

You see, you could postpone the confrontation by using all kinds of justifications. A common justification in this instance would be the comparison excuse, which may sound like this: "I'm not like a lotta my co-workers. They can't even fit into their clothes."

Sometimes, we'll just lay the responsibility elsewhere: "I started putting on a few pounds ever since my divorce."

Other times, we'll resist by openly objecting to the obvious, as in the case of a tremendous Oscar-winning American actress who would simply brush her obesity aside by saying, "I'm just a big girl!"

We may do or say anything to resist confronting ourselves, until the "they" I mentioned really touch a nerve. And then, suddenly and thank heavens, a sixth sense kicks in. There's a crack in your armor of hopelessness.

Soon, that crack begins to open wider, and vulnerability lays itself bare. That's when that sixth sense begins its free reign, informing you this is a call to arms.

And, most importantly, as you shed the lie, it informs you that you have the power to effectuate relief.

Boom!

Breakthrough!

MINDSET ADJUSTMENT!

This displays the power of a *magic moment* and its ability to affect mindset in a most profound and positive way. That's what a magic moment did for Mo'Nique, the aforementioned actress.

She revealed on a late-night talk show how she experienced that magic moment when her husband said, "That's too much weight. I want you around for a lifetime, and that's not healthy."

It touched a nerve, and it was worth a lot more than the weight she later shed. Eventually, she went down to under two hundred pounds after weighing as much as three hundred pounds.

She decided to save her life. Here's what she said: "It was at that moment that I went through guilt, I went through shame, because of my size—because I never felt love like that before.

"...I have a son who is twenty-three, but I also have a son who is nine. And we have twins who are seven. I want to meet their children. I want to be able to play with their children. I don't want to be a burden on my family due to self-neglect... I was fortunate to watch my grandmother play with my children. I want to be in the same position."

Yes, our lives are made up of interconnecting stories, many of which have the power to transform us beyond measure.

That one magic moment had that kind of effect, and it became a moving and inspirational interconnecting story for many others. Mo'Nique has even turned her attention to helping others with their weight-loss problems.

What bears stressing is, whenever we're moved by an inspirational story, foot-dragging can cause giant opportunities to pass us by.

In other words, to make the best of what we're experiencing, we need to take action before the feeling dissipates. Hesitation can often lay waste to many splendid ideas and opportunities, leaving us later to ponder what might have been.

CHAPTER 9

Being in Touch

MY OWN MAGIC moments came, as you may recall, after my job-hunting misfires and as I lay in a hospital bed.

In fact, that painful experience after not being able to find a job was truly an example of how losing becomes winning. You see, that exercise I undertook to write down positive events—magic moments—became second nature to me.

It became a habit that morphed into something else.

I wanted a way to keep these events alive. Now, every magic moment I come across—and there are many during the course of a day—becomes fodder for a private greeting card collection I created many years ago. But that's a story for another day!

It was the habit of noting these events that primed me not only to instinctively recall that incident with the baby climbing the stairs of a brownstone, but also to be inspired by that moment to create a little magic for myself.

In addition, it was a recollection that began to put me in touch with an innate part of myself—the same part that has taken its leave of so many of us.

Yes, that negative mindset took ahold of me for a short while after my hip surgery. It took that image of a baby to renew my spirit and inform (or remind) me I had it in me to undertake a kick-ass rehabilitation.

That is how far-reaching the ripples from a pebble dropped in a pond can be.

Suddenly, the birth of my children took on new meaning. Suddenly, this book came into view. Suddenly, I found a new way to pass on some value.

Not only did this book become a reality, but along with it arrived a reason.

You see, my own struggles with poor mindset and then my own breakthrough launched me on a new path to inspire others to action. The birth of my children solidified this, because watching them grow has sharpened the default instinct restarted by my exercise of taking note of life's little nuggets.

I call it a "default instinct" because curiosity is a feature built into every single one of us. It's the kind of instinct that often will drive parents crazy, as their child clambers up and over things to reach object after object that has captured his or her attention.

We've all been there, but, for the most part, we have left this part of ourselves way back in the distance, so we miss how significant these moments can be.

And so, yes, as my children retool my instincts, they continue to supply me with some pretty awesome magic moments, many of which I will share in the next chapters.

I am sure you will find they can awaken our senses in some pretty profound ways, as well as illuminate the path that has, from the very beginning, always been our roadmap to the way forward.

CHAPTER 10

Persistence and Determination are Omnipotent

PAIN!

There is no one among us who has not had an intimate experience with pain. Up close and personal.

And while it may not be a constant, at some point or other it becomes life's companion, and a familiar one at that.

That is why we experience the same emotional swings that a good movie can inspire.

Since the birth of my son, Kiichi, and daughter, Aiko, I have found myself in many real-life movies.

One in particular causes me to wince and then chuckle, whenever I think about it.

On his third morning out of the womb, Kiichi remained in a deep sleep for most of the day, having been sedated for circumcision. Needless to say, when he awoke after his long period of shuteye, he was famished and dove into feasting on mother's milk.

This soon necessitated a diaper change. His doting dad was more than happy to do the honors. But I quickly realized that providing relief would not be as easy as I'd thought.

In fact, it was more like executing a rescue, because, as it turned out, the gauze applied by the nurse after circumcision was fully stuck to my son's little wound.

Yes, *stuck*!

Needless to say, this early bout of pain was not pleasant for him. Despite my ginger approach to the task at hand, Kiichi's every scream pierced me like a dagger. Finally, thankfully, the gauze became unglued.

And before re-dressing the wound, I made sure to slather it generously with Vaseline.

Shortly thereafter, when we arrived home from the hospital, I realized there was more to this real-life movie, which continued to unfold as soon as I placed my son on the changing table for another diaper change.

After what he had endured, I was so overjoyed to see him happily lying on his back, kicking the air nonchalantly without a care in the world.

Then, suddenly, he did care. Just like that!

Yes, as soon as I loosened his diaper, his happy-go-lucky attitude went right out the window. Next, his eyes—those little windows to his soul—bulged with realization. He let out a knowing scream, which amounted to, you guessed it, "*Not again!*"

It hardly mattered that tending to the wound was a snap, this time around. Kiichi was prepared to take drastic action against this continued incursion.

And he did.

Before he did so, it actually crossed my mind that he would. He refused any food for about twenty-four hours. Yes, that little brain was whirring, and he had actually put two and two together:

No food in, no going to the bathroom.

No going to the bathroom, no diaper change.

Then, he abruptly abandoned his hunger strike, but only because he had to. It simply became a bit much to handle.

That's when he stuffed himself into blimpdom, passed out, tumbling from my arms onto his face, and, very soon thereafter, erupted like a volcano in his diaper.

Call it trauma or call it fear, that built-in instinct can make persistence and determination omnipotent. As Calvin Coolidge reminded us in discussing the importance of persistence and determination, *"Nothing in the world can take the place of perseverance."*

CHAPTER 11

Finding a Way to Overcome

HOW MANY TIMES have we done it?

If we're really being truthful, we'll call it what it is.

The "it" I'm referring to is what amounts to throwing our hands up in air. It's what I did when I retreated from the world after my terrible job-hunting experience.

At the time, I allowed myself to gift-wrap it all into a convenient explanation, one that pitted me against "them"—all those others who meant me no good.

But now I know better than that. As much as I hate to admit it, the simple explanation is I had thrown my hands up in the air and quit.

Yes, *quit*! Let's call a spade a spade. This was high-level quitting in typical "no más" terms.

And that's really saying a lot, because it was the kind of high-level quitting that made "no más" a household term, after boxing great Roberto Duran simply quit, uttering the words "no más"–"no more"–right in the middle of one of the most iconic fights in pugilistic history.

Now, in spite of his spectacular accomplishments, Duran is remembered more for quitting than for being one of the most terrifying fighters to have entered the ring. Of course, Duran's case is an extreme one, because of who he was. While my "no más" moment would never make the front pages, it was no less significant.

That's because, every time we throw our hands up in the air and retreat from life, our psyche takes a direct hit. Duran's psyche took a massive hit, and he would later regret that moment, as "no más" became integrated into pop-culture history, to live on forever.

Of course, what really matters is this: Finding a way to overcome.

That is what Duran did. Through perseverance, he again became a champion.

It is that same perseverance legendary NFL coach Vince Lombardi alluded to when he said:

> *Getting knocked down is part of life, and if you stay down, you're not going to get very far. Getting back up is the key to success in all areas of life, business, finances, relationships, and health.*

> *There are surely moments in your life where you've been knocked down, but you found a way to pick yourself back up and carry on. Use these memories as a highlight reel to help you get back up more quickly the next time you get knocked down. It's easy to do it again when you've confirmed you've done it before.*

Yes, memories. I have my own and lot, lot more.

From my front-row seat, I am reminded, time and again, of Lombardi's inspirational words.

That's because that front-row seat is an invaluable perch. From it, I have had access to an unlimited highlight reel that reveals countless instances of true grit—persistence and determination—that is nothing short of the will to win.

CHAPTER 12

The Will to Win

THE LOMBARDI TEAMS, the Green Bay Packers, were known for their heart power—their non-quitting spirit.

Yes, he was a coach, but he was in the business of building character. And today, it is common to hear a winning coach refer to his team as having "character."

One of the most profound Lombardi utterances is a mere three words, but it remains an enduring metaphor:

"Inches make champions."

Of course, he was drawing on his experiences on the football field, where inches can, at times, be the difference between winning and losing. The thing is, he was well positioned to watch his players battle, time and again, when they gave all they had to move the ball inches at a time.

Lombardi would often equate football with life. You see, if you can give your all, even if it's just to gain inches, no mountain will seem high enough to dissuade you.

I have witnessed a similar kind of perseverance in my children's development. It is that innate discipline at the highest level that fosters the habit of always reaching higher and higher to overcome, in spite of obstacles.

I recall one struggle from the depths— a grind. It was a fight to move not inches, but maybe just *an* inch, maybe less. Sometimes, zero. But you fight on, because it's about this: Never giving ground.

This is what giving your all looks like.

Just think for a moment. When you wake up each day, you would like to get from here to there, but it means struggling to move even an inch. I'm sure you'd agree those are bad days.

But wait! They may not be bad after all!

I am thinking about tummy time, those first occasions when I placed my kids on their stomachs. Almost every time I put them down on their stomachs, they were looking for a win. With little faces contorted, nostrils flaring, and mouths quivering, they would flail their arms, never failing to give it their all. Their screams seemed to will them on.

And yes, they did begin to progress inch by inch, always instinctively reaching for the next challenge. Once they beat the first challenge, it would deliver a boost to their winning spirit and urge them on with enthusiasm. Inch by inch began to add up. And suddenly, they'd be looking for more.

And "more" could turn out to be breathtaking! Like the day I was caught by surprise when, as Kiichi sat playing with a toy, he suddenly appeared to be losing his balance.

I was sure he was about to fall but, before I could comprehend exactly what was happening, he rolled three times in rapid succession.

Then, Aiko executed this new method of travel with such deft proficiency, it was as if she had been equipped with a GPS that prevented her from banging into the sides of her crib.

The remarkable thing is, the inch-by-inch struggle is how we all can bring each successive milestone into view. This includes you! It's exactly how we did it way, way back when, as infants.

This is the same inch-by-inch struggle that made so much sense to me when I recalled little Lindsay Guerrero climbing up those stairs. Inch by inch swiftly added up, and I was soon walking on air.

So, if you find yourself dragging your feet, apply this strategy. In other words, start somewhere!

Don't look at the whole staircase!

Take Lombardi's words to heart! Paste them on your wall!

Look forward to those inches adding up! It's what eventually gets us across the goal line to burst into the end zone.

Call it what you may—grit, persistence, determination, character. But Lombardi couldn't have said it better:

"Inches make champions."

CHAPTER 13

It's Not Whether You Get Knocked Down But Whether You Get Up

– Vince Lombardi

CHAMPIONS DEFINE their presence on the field of play through courage. Being courageous is how we develop the heart of a champion.

Having the heart of a champion means getting knocked down and having the courage to get back up after being flattened yet still remain disciplined enough to have that singular focus on your goal.

I would like to suggest you do something now. *Really* do this:

Take the time to watch kids.

Do it with a different eye than you normally would, and you will see how they display the heart of a champion regularly, as they move from one stage in their development to the next.

I cannot tell you how many times, as my kids began to learn how to sit, their developing muscles betrayed them, and they capsized backward with a thud and burst into screams.

And you guessed it: They never stayed down.

They would, however long it took, right themselves and resume fingering those little hanging objects in their baby gym. Even when bruised and bloodied, they would not be deterred. And, as cuts and bruises go, one moment stands out.

One day, when my daughter, Aiko, was about two years old, she had her own bloody mishap. To put things into perspective, if you climb, there's always a risk of falling.

She had fallen a few times while climbing in and out of her crib. And, yes, she'd popped right back up to pick up where she'd left off.

Then one day, in what had become routine for her, she clambered onto a bed. But this time, she lost her balance and toppled, headfirst, onto the nearby side table.

However, even with a nasty gash above one of her eyes, her resilience took center stage, and she hopped right back on the horse. She never, even for a moment, became gun-shy about climbing.

In fact, not long after, I had to turn and quickly grab my phone when she said, "Picture, Papa. picture!"

There she was, standing tiptoe on the windowsill balanced on one leg, with her other leg stretched up to the top rail in a near-180-degree split. And she was facing her brother, Kiichi, who had assumed the exact same position.

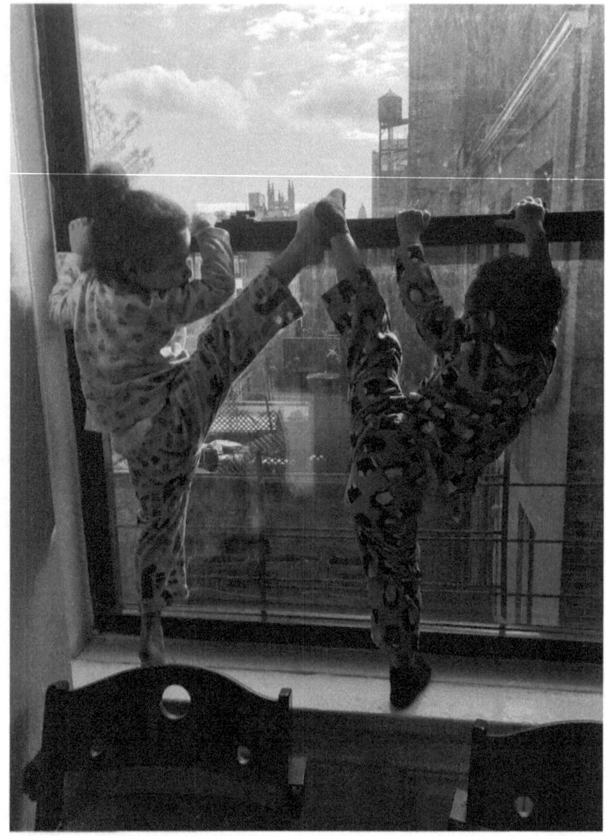

Resilience taking center stage

From my front-row seat, I have never seen such consistency of risk-taking tomd then picking one's self back up again.

By this measure, I've watched both of my kids overcome adversity to become champions many times over, sometimes during the course of a day, with disciplined efforts that bordered on comedy.

If, as Lombardi once said, "There's something good in all of us that yearns for discipline," this next story demonstrates a remarkable disciplined effort by a ten-month-old who decided to take the road less traveled, when he figured crawling was a bit mundane. That particular road less traveled led straight to an immobile toy car he liked to crawl inside.

This car was Kiichi's favorite, because it had bells and whistles that played some pretty catchy tunes. It became his home away from home. He would yank the door open, crawl in, pull himself into the seat, and start pressing buttons that set off a musical extravaganza.

Soon, however, he decided it was time to make things a bit more interesting. Still not yet walking, he one day felt ambitious and elected to court adversity. Who said we need our legs under us for a successful climb?

Rules are made to be broken, and he would simply just buck the rules. Why should he continue opening doors when he could just as well climb over them?

So, one day, he entered through one of the car's little doors but then decided to exit by climbing over the next. As he attempted his climb, however, he toppled headfirst onto the floor.

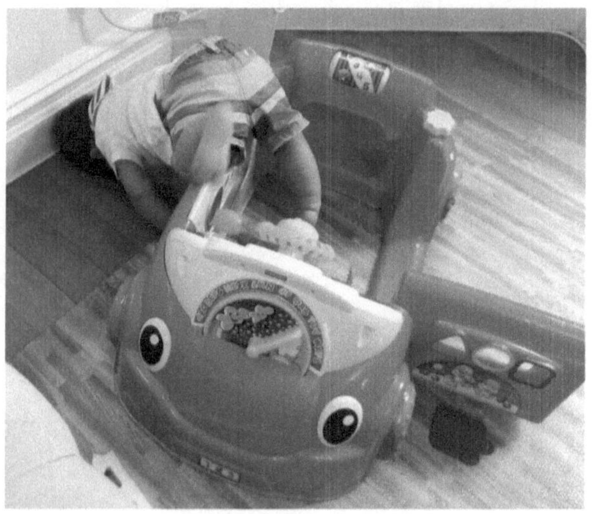

Commitment!

Through his disciplined effort, he did keep trying, though, even after falling on his head again and again.

This was a demonstration of a basic law of life: Success has a price, and if you don't pay the price, you can't win.

This was *commitment*!

And guess what?

My son's will, which refused to give in, eventually won out.

CHAPTER 14

The Commitment in a Smile

IT'S ONE THING to be told you're behaving like a child, but it's quite another to be childlike. That's because being childlike may not be a bad idea after all.

Did you ever notice how, when a young child smiles how, there is no mistaking, it comes from deep inside? From toe to head. With no pretention, no phoniness.

It is a smile that seems to radiate from every fiber of that child's body.

That is what a winning smile looks like.

It's this kind of smile that, according to research, reduces stress within us and helps to generate more positive emotions.

Estimates have it that, on average, babies smile about 200 times a day, which is why, experts say, we often feel happier around them. And there is no explanation needed as to why the smiley face is one of the most-used symbols anywhere. **There is just no mistaking the power and energy a smile emanates.**

Imagine smiling from deep inside 200 times per day! This takes commitment, putting your all into every smile.

It was this same commitment I saw in my kids, starting from the moment they clawed and struggled on their stomach, trying to move just an inch or less. The energy and enthusiasm of commitment were what propelled them over obstacles and from one milestone to the next.

Their approach underlines this basic fact: Once we've achieved a measure of success, it stokes our furnace and readies us for further challenges.

Success lights a fire and triggers something *good* inside of us. I saw that *good* inside the day my son jumped up from the toilet, looked back, displayed that emotional currency of a smile, and ran off, fists in the air, shouting triumphantly, "I did it! *I did it!*"

Day after day, he had worked his heart out, trying to do this. Then, suddenly, his finest hour arrived. Potty training was another challenge he had faced down, leading him to more confidence gained and a boost to tackle more adversity head-on.

Adversity plays a huge role in growth. It is a vital fuel for greatness.

The journey from being a baby on its back to a toddler running off, pumping his fists in the air to claim victory with a winning smile is remarkable— nothing short of greatness. It is a journey of incredible wins fraught with adversity. That is why victory can be so intoxicating.

I have seen what that adversity engendered in a couple of toddlers who often climbed to the highest perch and raised their arms above their heads to proclaim, "I am the king of the world!" before launching themselves into the air.

Then, over and over, they would hit the floor with a thump. But they'd gather themselves up for one last jump before I'd be forced to call a halt to their giddy madness.

Yes, adversity is why the thrill of victory can be so sweet. It is something that inspires us toward that moving goalpost.

Call their giddy madness kids' play, but, as they go through the developmental process, children demonstrate a commitment that is truly special. They play with their heart and every fiber of their body.

They'll have it no other way. It's the only way.

Through bumps and bruises, they will cry at the top of their lungs, only to reassume default mode and regain their enthusiasm, picking back up right where they left off.

Yes, it's that enthusiasm that makes my kids stand in a chair with a smile of commitment, fists waving, as if they've hit gold, and chanting with excitement, "I'm getting big! I'm getting big!"

CHAPTER 15

Hitting Gold and Then Some

IT HAS HAD far-reaching effects. But it was, after all, just a thought!

But was it really just that?

Well, it inspired a smile. And that inspired a feeling of hope. Then hope turned to "yes, you can." And "yes, you can" inspired a feeling of triumph." That feeling of triumph planted a knowing seed that I could overcome. And that knowing feeling caused my blood to pulsate.

As that pulsating blood pumped to a drumming crescendo, it caused something to rise up inside of me.

So, yes, maybe I should have stood in the middle of my hospital bed and waved my fists around like a kid who'd reached another milestone, but, after all, my first walk to nowhere had just begun its slow transformation to somewhere. The ripple effect led to a place I could never have imagined.

It was like a pebble dropped in a pond, causing a ripple that travels way beyond where it started and reverberates across a great distance and span of time.

As I write this, I remain aware that that ripple is ongoing because, once set in motion, its ability to transform is beyond incredible.

When the thought of a baby climbing on all fours up the stairs of a brownstone entered my mind and moved me to action, I could never have foreseen how far that inspirational thought would take me. I certainly could never have imagined this book would be part of the equation.

That equation involved a change of perspective in ways I could not foresee or anticipate. For one, it fueled my rehabilitation from the get-go.

And as that fire burned within to get started, I was sure of this: I would not be limiting myself to just being able to get back on my feet so I could take walks and maybe go hiking.

No, siree!

Not after being able to effortlessly propel myself through the air, making one full revolution before striking a heavy bag with a kick! The sky would always continue to be the limit for me.

I was determined to get back to anything and everything I'd done before. And I did!

So much so that the amazing Dr. Edwin Su, who headed the bionic-like nuts-and-bolts effort that put me back together at New York's Hospital For Special Surgery, acknowledged his part in the ripple effect, when, after my last follow-up visit a year later, he said, "I feel like I see you every day. I use your pictures in my lectures."

The thing is, those lectures often reach dozens of overseas medical personnel via closed-circuit television.

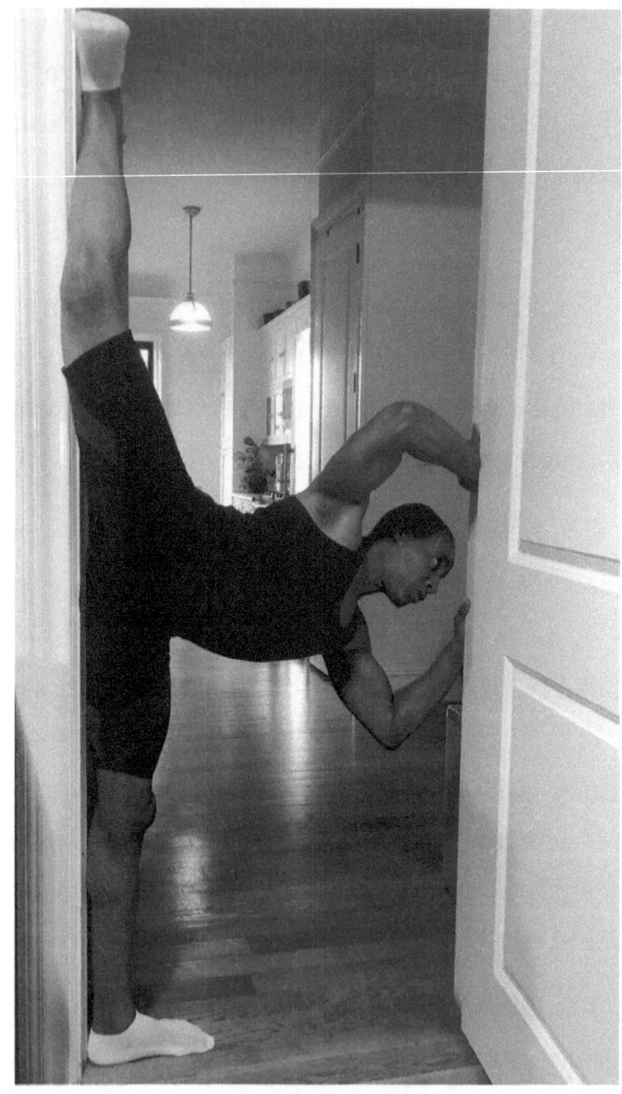

Reclaiming lost ability

That pebble in the pond continues to be instructional on how a ripple in life can have far-reaching effects. For one, it opened my eyes in a special way after my children made their dramatic entry. Yes, with their birth alone, I struck gold.

But then there was the "and then some." You see, while their entry made me an immensely appreciative parent, at the same time it offered a great vantage point from my capacity as a fitness coach.

It set in motion a unique vision and perspective, born of the fact that I could now harness amazingly valuable information as I watched my children's physical development.

CHAPTER 16

The Extraordinarily Efficient Traveling Gym

HOW MANY TIMES has an unfortunate wrinkle made you sit up and pay attention?

That's the beautiful thing about adversity. I truly believe it was the driving force that made me sit up and pay attention in ways I never would have, otherwise.

It drove me to continue reaching for the stars—to see how much further I could take my body past what I had achieved in my physical recovery.

That is when, like a child homes in on a new discovery, a lightbulb went off that captured my curiosity. Then, a clear picture came into view of why I had lost the wind in my sails and ended up dragging myself around in pain.

The result?

I became a better fitness coach. While getting myself back on my feet and in shape was a great goal, it wasn't good enough. I now had an eye on developing programs that worked for me—programs based on specific functional body movements.

These were the same foundational building blocks at work that piloted my kids from lying on their backs to turning over, to rolling and crawling, standing and walking, running, jumping, and everything else in between.

This was the *forgotten blueprint* that not only put the spring back in my step but also had me tipping my hat, as I cultivated more of an eye to how most of us could get back to basics and avoid or banish some pretty common debilitating ailments, like plantar fasciitis and patella tendonitis.

The basics could be reduced to this concept: Doing what has to be the best exercise there is. But chances are and as science has found, if you are like most people, you are not doing *this*. And if you're not doing it, you may be saddled with one or more ailments because of this neglect.

What I'm about to tell you is something you've heard before. But what you may not know is you can do this and reap physical benefits all day, without setting foot in a gym.

Please hold that thought and let me ask you this: Have you ever watched a toddler squat to the ground to retrieve something?

If you have, it may not have occurred to you that you were being treated to a perfect example of *how to bend*.

And if you've ever been taught to bend properly, you may not actually know just how much of a golden nugget this is.

If you'd like to experience the exhilaration of getting back to basics, here is a friendly challenge that could help things come together smoothly for you. I recommend you use a mirror to practice what I'm about to tell you.

Remember this: Bending over from your hips or waist deposits hundreds of pounds of pressure on your lower back. With our poor bending habits, it is no surprise that, according to one study, "low back pain is the leading cause of activity limitation and work absence throughout much of the world."

For the dozens of times you have to bend each day (the estimate is in the *hundreds*), do the following:

1. Keep your heels down firmly. Shift your weight back, so it is supported by your heels.
2. Keep your bent knees over your feet and not jutting forward. In other words, if you look down and cannot see your toes because your knees are in the way, you are practicing a common habit that will surely cause knee pain.
3. Keep your hips tucked under as you lower down, just enough to where you are able to keep your back straight. As you bend, be sure not to stick your butt out behind you.

"Yes," you may be thinking. "I've heard this before." But this time, think about all the bending we do, large and small!

We bend at the file cabinet, bend to pick up something from the ground, bend to pet the cat or the dog, bend at the wash basin, bend to open drawers, bend to tie our laces, bend to vacuum the floor, and on and on in daily life.

And the rub is, most of us bend incorrectly. Over time, this can result in a domino-effect-like cascade of debilitating injuries, which, if left unchecked, can even affect our ability to breathe, if we have developed an unsightly acute forward head posture.

And, of course, there's the gym. Yes, the gym!

Many times, this is where you'll see people doing toe touches, crunching forward, and lifting weights by bending forward, positioning themselves in ways that can cause injury.

Then, finally, to add insult to injury, they will bend over incorrectly to pick up their gym bag and head home!

Are you skeptical about the merits of good bending? Try, with focus and good technique, to bend correctly for an entire day. I guarantee you, by day's end, your legs and core will feel as if you'd had a strenuous workout at the gym, complete with natural stretching for your Achilles tendons, hamstrings, and calves.

Of course, this is a basic revisiting of what a developing child does, but it is the rock-solid foundation for preventing or managing a host of potentially sidelining maladies.

And you know what has been said about practice. Yes, it makes perfect—especially in this case, considering that nature's prescription from the very beginning has equipped us all with an extraordinarily efficient traveling gym.

CHAPTER 17

Take a Bow and Tip Your Hat to a Fatty Example!

IF WE ARE LOOKING for a great example of something, it is a good bet we will look to the best. Every time.

It makes perfect sense. Why would we want anything less?

But, sometimes, looks can be deceiving. How about striving to look like a sumo wrestler? No?

Of course, with a chuckle, you're thinking, "Those guys are obese! Who would want to look like that?"

I wouldn't want to look like that, either. But, with optimum glucose, cholesterol, and triglyceride levels, through tremendous amounts of exercise, they escape those well-known maladies associated with excess weight (unlike the rest of us).

Of course, neither would I want to look like my kids did on their first days of life.

But, wait a minute!

I *did* look like them once, since babies are born with a higher percentage of body fat than any other species. Yes, at birth, humans are the fattest species, with a whopping fifteen percent body fat.

And these little sumo wrestlers we give birth to continue to grow fatter, peaking at about twenty-five percent body fat between four and nine months of age. After that point, they normally start to thin out. For myself, however, besides being no good for health, I would find it quite uncomfortable to carry around all that giggly fat.

Notwithstanding the foregoing, if you are part of the fat-bashing battalion, you may need to dislodge yourself from the ranks. The truth is, when we are discussing getting into shape, fat is often the boogeyman. However, this is what needs to be highlighted:

If you are in search of your best health (which I assume my readers would be), sensible nutrition is a must. In this chapter, *fat* occupies a place of honor, because no food that is so crucial to overall health has also been so vilified.

You see, fat is absolutely necessary. Avoiding it is not a good idea, especially since fat is the way we and all other mammals store energy.

In other words, if you're looking for the best demonstration of why fat can be so important for good health, you just have to look in the mirror. Take a bow and tip your hat to this fatty example: You!

Back on your first day alive, you, too, were born with all that fat in order to make up for any shortage of energy or nutrition. And you continued to store a lot of it, because without it, growth or brain development would have been seriously impeded.

I am sure you are understanding my point. The ability to process what I've explained on this page is due, in large part, to fat! The fatty truth is our brains are composed of sixty percent fat, and they cannot work correctly without it.

The bottom line is this: fueling ourselves with fat can, in addition to other benefits, not only keep the rest of us healthy, but also help stave off brain diseases, while, at the same time, having positive effects on learning and memory.

That said, this is no endorsement to eat fat indiscriminately. Rather, it is a call to learn how to use it wisely—and to your advantage.

So, I'll say this. Whether you're looking for that all-round healthy you, the high-performance body of an athlete, or simply want to shed some pounds, fat could be your magic bullet.

If some sixty to seventy percent of your diet consists of fat, your body will have to binge on fat for fuel. Hence, the scientific logic that you need fat to burn fat.

This involves limiting your carbohydrates and ingesting wholesome protein, low-starch vegetables, and high-quality fats such as eggs, avocado, cheese, nuts, and let's not forget butter.

Your magic bullet will also enable you to absorb fat-soluble vitamins, along with powerful disease-fighting anti-oxidants that protect us against free radicals, which are constantly invading our bodies to accelerate aging.

Armed with your magic bullet, the rule of thumb would be this:

- ➢ Eat protein and fats when you're less active or sedentary.
- ➢ Eat protein and carbohydrates when you're active.

For a comprehensive explanation, please email me at rocketfuelcoach@gmail.com.

CHAPTER 18

That High-Octane Rocket Fuel

REVISITING SO MANY of my experiences with my kids was not just a personal exercise. In many ways, this is also *your* story.

The common denominator here is that built-in propellant, a type of *high-octane rocket fuel* that launched each of us along the same developmental path, starting from the very beginning of our lives.

You and I have traveled the same road as my son, who jumped from the toilet yelling, "I did it! I did it!" If a picture is worth a thousand words, his fist pumps said it all.

These moments remind us that "inches make champions" and that, deep within, we still carry what took us from lying on our back to eventually standing on our own two feet.

Earlier, I mentioned this book is about rediscovering a big truth—a truth that continues to elude many of us; one that needs constant reinforcement.

It is simply this: We come equipped with all we need to succeed.

Nowhere is that more evident than in our spectacular and eventful march, as children. Yet, in our eventful march as adults, our struggles often arrest and defeat us, separating us from those winning childhood years, while reducing us to seeing the glass as half empty too often—sometimes even completely empty, as in my case on that frightful day in the hospital.

It bears remembering that our lives are made up of interconnecting stories and events, many of which you could very well call your own. It was one of those *magic moments* I mentioned that touched a nerve in me, as I lay in my hospital bed. It was one of those events that touched a nerve in me when I wallowed in hopelessness, after my futile efforts at finding a job.

Be habitual in taking note, and you will begin to appreciate the magic of these moments, just as I did, when I found myself in the middle of one of them. I have bottled it in my memory and gone back to it many times, in order to inspire myself to action.

That moment came one evening in the bitter cold, as I dashed along West 14th Street in New York City, hardly relishing the short couple of blocks to the subway.

"Sir, can you please help me across the street?" came a woman's voice. Familiar to anyone who loves old movies, as I do, this voice reminded me of the aged, silver-haired acting legend, Katharine Hepburn.

As I offered a hand to support her, she steadfastly declined, even though her decades-old body had definitely seen its time.

"No, no," she answered with self-assured calm and determination. "Just walk beside me."

Then, as I waved traffic to a standstill, the light went through several changes before, at a snail's pace, we finally made it to the other side. It was a marathon of epic proportions, because it just may have been the slowest I had ever walked since learning to take my first steps.

For her, it was nothing short of a miraculous undertaking, with her body on its last legs—first by bus, then by subway from the far reaches of New Jersey, and now again to catch another bus on the other side of the street, in order to visit her daughter in a hospital in upper Manhattan.

On our epic walk across the street, she was able to tell me all this and more, which further underscores how slow a walk this was. However, despite its slow pace, it was nevertheless loaded with that *high octane* that lives within us.

CHAPTER 19

The Road Less Traveled

IT HAPPENED A LONG, long time ago, and yet it will continue to resonate into infinity. That is because it stresses something so crucial, if we are to continue growing or excelling.

Of course, the drumbeat to that resonance started way, way back in 1916, when Robert Frost's unforgettable poem "The Road Not Taken" was published. I'm willing to bet, while most of us cannot recall the entire poem, chances are we're familiar with these oft-repeated lines:

> *Two roads diverged in a wood, and I,*
> *I took the one less traveled by,*
> *And that has made all the difference.*

You may recall the account of my son taking the road less traveled, only to fall on his head continually, when attempting, over and over again, to climb out of his toy car, rather than leave through the door.

When I call this the road less traveled, I refer to something that happens to so many of us, myself included, as we leave the wonder years of childhood behind. The irony is, back then, this was whom we were—again and again taking the road less traveled.

That was normalcy.

And then, normalcy—no longer normal—took its leave, and a kind of reticence and even fear set in, robbing us of our dreams, until we no longer dream.

Yes, back when normalcy was second nature, we demonstrated remarkable persistence. But normalcy also highlighted something that Frost's poem so elegantly hammered home. The importance of taking risks.

Yes, if we are to grow or excel, taking risks is a must.

Of course, while taking risks to get to the next level is courageous, it hardly means the absence of fear. It means overcoming in spite of fear.

This replayed itself over and over again, as I watched my kids develop. It unnerved me to watch, with heart-pounding anxiety, as, with hesitancy and measured calculation, they attempted to jump from the sofa to the floor.

But I also have to admit, while my instinct was to be protective, I also recognized this is how real growth happens. There is no mistaking it: it is in taking that leap of faith that real growth happens for all of us.

It is what "made all the difference" for us as kids, and it is often what will make the difference for us as adults. No risk, no growth!

Of course, pulling the trigger—taking risks—is not without its pitfalls. But what can result from doing so can also be remarkably life-changing.

My son kept falling on his head. He risked this happening every time he attempted to climb out of that car, until it no longer happened. Suddenly, he found himself smoothly in the clear. Yes, that initial climb was a mere stepping stone to his tackling a higher mountain.

The thing is, we take unconscious risks every day throughout our life. How do we know every driver will adhere to that red light, the next time we cross the street? How do we know the next driver isn't suffering a heart attack? Or is not drunk or crazy?

The truth is we don't. Yet, unconsciously and at times carelessly, we step into the crosswalk, well before the approaching vehicle comes to a halt.

However, when it comes to challenging ourselves consciously by taking calculated risks, the crosswalk suddenly becomes foreign, and we falter, overtaken by fear.

How do I know that writing this book will make a shred of difference to anyone? I don't!

But what I do know is we once conquered fear, over and over, a long, long time ago, and we have the capacity to do it again, because of that *high octane* in our DNA—that *rocket fuel* that propelled my son time and again, even as he fell on his head.

Daring to go there again could be the best thing that ever happened to you.

CHAPTER 20

Get Used to Pressing the Default Button

AS WE COME TO the last chapter of this book, it is my hope you'll be inspired to press the default button as many times as needed, to unearth the kid in you.

The kid who, with resilience and enthusiasm and fueled by adversity, took risk after risk, fighting from one milestone to the next.

While much of this will surely be beyond our memory, there are truly uplifting human events around us every day that can help us to rekindle what once was second nature so long ago.

It is in that spirit that I urge you to try doing the following, something that could be positively life-changing: Get into the habit of bringing a notepad and pen with you. Make a note of all the positive events that come about to help you through your day. And do this until it becomes habit-forming.

Bear in mind, for something to become a habit, you will need to do it every day. One study, though not definitive, concluded that doing something for sixty-six days could make it habit-forming.

The truth is the length of time it takes will vary from person to person. You will know instinctively when it's automatic.

First, you will begin to notice the positive effect this noting of events has on your thinking. You will sense a calm about you, as you go through daily life.

And, yes, with calmness comes decreased stress levels. While there is good and bad stress, the bottom line is, according to one report, seventy-five to ninety percent of all doctor visits are for stress-related ailments and complaints.

What is certain is if you make it a habit to be curious, like a kid, you will instinctively find nuggets that'll enrich your life in unexpected ways. That is what happened to me some time ago, when I pressed the default button and unearthed a real *magic moment*— a nugget that was worth its weight in gold.

As I walked by a supermarket in New York City, I noticed a man in a discolored sailor cap standing next to an old bicycle that was as weather-beaten as he was.

With soft, searching, blue eyes, he asked matter-of-factly, "Can you please help me?"

Instinctively, I said, "Yes," without knowing how I'd be able to.

Next, he motioned me to step around his two-wheeled chariot. Then he asked that I, "very slowly and carefully" lift one of his legs over the seat and place it on the pedal. And he still had one more request. Could I pick up what felt like a lead-packed grocery bag and hang it on his handlebar?

After thanking me, he jarred me from my stupor by casually delivering the line of the day. "I'm only ninety-three-years young," he said, before steadily riding off.

He absolutely epitomized something my mother often said: "Where there's a will, there's a way."

That ninety-three-year-old could not get on his bicycle himself, but he found a way to forge through everyday tasks, even if he was on borrowed time.

As he rode away, I watched him slowly disappear, misty-eyed, and thought, "How's he ever going to get *off* that bicycle, especially with that heavy bag hanging from his handle bar? What happens if he has to stop for a red light?"

But I knew the answer: *The kid in him would find a way.*

And if he could, so could I.

That's how commitment becomes an engine that propels you. It becomes that *rocket fuel* that launches you.

What has happened to me since then reminds me of one of my favorite quotes, from W. H. Murray on the 1951 Scottish Himalayan Expedition.

"Until one is committed, there is hesitancy, the chance to draw back, always ineffectiveness, concerning all acts of initiative [and creation]. There is one elementary truth the ignorance of which kills countless ideas and splendid plans; that the moment one definitely commits oneself, then providence moves, too. All sorts of things occur to help one that would never otherwise have occurred."

Because of providence, I've become that man on the bicycle many times over, trusting that commitment makes things happen. Yet, instinctive commitment is no stranger; it's what propelled us from being a baby on its back to becoming incredible bipedal machines.

Commitment is how this book came about. It is also how I started my Internet coaching business, because I am committed to helping as many people as I can achieve their fitness goals. I could never have been as effective going door-to-door or camped out in a gym.

So, commitment as a fitness coach is what compels me to say: Your body is the greatest instrument you'll ever own, and the stress that can come about if you treat it poorly can overshadow everything else in your life.

So, if you feel yourself being neglectful, call on the kid in you, take the time to look around, and be assured you won't have to search very hard for your "man on the bicycle." He's always there to be found, because the universe is always conspiring to help.

Be inspired anew to be propelled to greatness by that *high-octane rocket fuel* already within you.

You'll feel better in everything you do!

MY GIFT TO YOU

I'M PASSIONATE ABOUT the strategies in this book, because they've worked for me. I'd like to give you a gift for reading this far.

It's based on the same strategies that worked for us all, when we were kids.

I'd like to help you recapture the same passion that propelled you to greatness many times over—from lifting up your head to turning over on your back to rolling, crawling, and finally walking. I'm sure you'll agree, it took the right ingredients to accomplish all that.

So, I'm offering you a free weight-loss program to thank you for reading this book. It will show you how to tap into what is already inside of you by putting into action some of the same strategies that have worked for me.

Simply email me here:

RocketfuelCoach@gmail.com

ACKNOWLEDGMENTS

THANKS TO MY MOTHER, Icodel Tomlinson, for fertilizing that seed in my brain when you said, "You should write a book." Mom, you're my inspiration!

Thanks to my sister, Yvette Tomlinson, for believing in me a very long time ago—long before I even gave a thought to doing this.

Thanks to my wife, Risa Morisada who, in willing me on and picking up the slack, thought I had a story to tell. And my two amazing angels, Kiichi and Aiko, who in teaching me a thing or two have been constant reminders of what it means to just be.

Thank you, Lindsay Guerrero, who, with a special memory, willed me to climb some stairs after I left my hospital bed.

To AJ Mihrzad and Pat Pilla, for creating that winning environment that lit a fire under me to finally get on with it and write this book.

Thank you, Sarah Andrew, for allowing little Lindsay into my life way back when.

Thank you to Betty Zimmer, for telling me in so many ways that commitment is what makes things happen.

And thank you to everyone who, in crossing my path, has inspired me in some way.

And Let's Not Forget

Last *but by no means least*, as you close this book, please save a thought for the millions of kids who are unable to simply just be. Yes, the cancer of poverty continues to rob millions of their potential, as they grow up without family and community structures to nurture and protect them.

So, as we nurture our own, let's not forget the millions who go without.

It behooves us, because the alternative would be to turn our backs on the incredibly promising foundation on which our world sits.

ABOUT THE AUTHOR

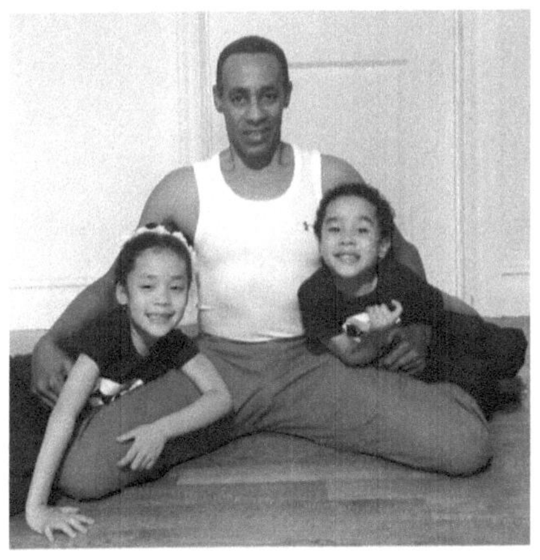

PHILLIP TOMLINSON is a fitness expert and experienced athlete, with a Master of Science Degree from Columbia University. A former track and field competitor and soccer player, he also holds a black belt in karate.

Phillip has been a medical editor and an award-winning reporter who has covered a range of topics, from science and technology to diet, exercise, and sports injuries. His experience in body movement resulted in the BodinSync fitness system, which utilizes compound exercises to complement the body's natural inclinations.

To learn more about BodinSync, please visit www.bodinsync.com.